Taking Control of Your Health

A Healthcare Guide for Patients

Taking Control of Your Health

A Healthcare Guide for Patients

Shanna F. McCoy

Printed in the United States of America

First Printing, 2018

ISBN: 978-1-947656-76-5

ISBN10: 1947656767

Butterfly Typeface Publishing
PO Box 56193
Little Rock, AR 72215

www.butterflytypeface.com

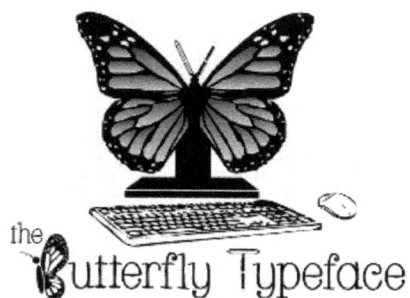

the
Butterfly Typeface

For my Father

"Either you let life live you

or you can choose to live life

to the fullest.

Which do you choose?

When striving to reach your full potential,

always strive for the best.

If you can't reach the moon,

at least try to hang with the stars."

Table of Contents

Acknowledgments

First, I would like to give a special acknowledgment to the Creator,
for blessing me with the ability to put my thoughts on paper.

Thank you to my African/Caribbean ancestors
who were enslaved against their will,
this book is dedicated to you all, your 4th generation daughter.

I would like to give an acknowledgement to my family, both my African/Native American ancestors, both known and unknown, who made special sacrifices, and laid a very strong foundation of the woman I have become:

Thank you to Mr. Greene and Mrs. Elizabeth Reynolds (aka Reynolos),
who were both members of the Chickasaw/Choctaw/ Cherokee and Mississippi Band of Choctaw and Creek Nation.

Thank you to my great grandparents, Mr. and Mrs. John Rollins Jr.
and my great grandmother, Mrs. Mattie Reynolos Rollins
(member of the Chickasaw & Choctaw/ Cherokee/Creek Nation).

Thank you to my grandparents,
Mr. and Mrs. John and Estella Rollins.

Thank you to my friends:
Ms. Cassandra Williamson, Ms. Gina Scott, and Ms. Street.

Thank you to Mr. Lee Booye (my cab driver), who gave advice
and drove me to every event in Arkansas.

Thank you Mr. Larry D. Freeman and Ms.Vivian Carroll, childhood friends,

thanks for your wisdom and advice.

Thank you to Mr. Danny Ray Cephas for being by my side.

You were a part of my history.

There will never be any one who can take your place.

Now you can rest in peace.

Thank you to my siblings, it has been an amazing ride.

Love you all.

A big thank you to *Mr. St. Louis* and his family.

Finally, to my parents Mr. W.C. Rollins and Mrs. Carrie McCoy-King,

thank you for giving me wings to fly in the face of adversity.

You gave me strength and courage to become greater than myself.

To my mother, thank you for having a strong will power, and dedication,

to ensure that one day all your hard work would pay off.

Preface

Taking Control of Your Health, A HealthCare Guide for Patients provides a place for patients to:

- Document How You Feel Daily
- Maintain A Current Listing Of All Medication
- Organize Your Health Concerns
- Prepare Questions For Your Healthcare Team
- Retrieve Medical Records
- Transfer Medical Records
- Track Appointments

The template documents provided in this book can help you to effectively and efficiently communicate our concerns to your healthcare team and allow written documentation for family who may need to assist.

Introduction

There are some diseases that don't seem to get the attention I think they deserve. Then there are those that we are all too familiar with.

Whatever your disease, I know this guide will be helpful to you and those who may be assisting you on your medical journey.

Along with your loved ones, we want to encourage you in your fight.

Use these templates and be inspired to add others that may be helpful as well. Purchasing this book is another step in taking control of your health.

There is power in participating in your care!

As a person who is outliving Cerebral Palsy and living with an inoperable brain tumor, I know firsthand the importance of participating in your care.

My encouragement to you is this:

> "And behold, they brought to him a man sick of the palsy, lying on a bed and Jesus seeing their faith said unto the sick of the palsy; Son be of good cheer; thy sins be forgiven thee. And, behold, certain of the scribes said within themselves, This man blasphemeth. And Jesus knowing their thoughts said, wherefore think ye evil in your hearts? For whether is easier, to say, Thy sins be forgiven thee; or to say, Arise, and walk? But that ye may know that the Son of man hath power on earth to forgive sins, (then saith he to the sick of the palsy,) Arise, take up they bed, and go unto thine house. And he arose and departed to this house. But when the multitudes saw it, they marveled, and glorified God, which had given such power unto men." **Matthew 9:2-8 (KJV)**

Medical Records Release Letter

Date   _____

Business Name   _____

Mailing Address   _____

City, State, Zip   _____

Dear Sir or Madam:

I am writing to request a copy of my medical records.

I am currently a patient of Dr. _____. Enclosed is a signed *Authorization to Release Medical Records*.

If there is a charge for copying the records, please submit a statement with the records and I will remit payment upon receipt of the records. Please contact me at the address below if you have any questions or need additional information.

I can also be reached by phone at _____. Thank you for your attention to this matter.

Sincerely,

Your Name

Your address

City, State, Zip

Enclosure

Authorization to Release Medical Records

(1) **Patient Information**

Name _____

SSN _____

Date of Birth _____

Address _____

(2) **Authorization for Release**

I hereby authorize _____ of _____

_____, _____ _____ to
release, disclose, and deliver the medical information described below to:

Authorized Recipient:

_____

_____

_____

(3) **Specific Authorization.** I specifically authorize the release of all medical information relating to the above-named patient including but not limited to the following categories protected by state of federal law: (1) substance abuse (drug or alcohol) treatment; (2) Mental health treatment; and (3) HIV-AIDS related information, if such information is contained in the records. This request includes any reports, correspondence, test results, and any other information contained in the records, whether generated by the authorized provider or another entity.

I do not give permission for any other use of redisclosure of this information.

Date _____

Signature _____

(4) **Redisclosure**. This release does not authorize redisclosure of medical information beyond the limits of this consent. The recipient of this information is prohibited from using the information for other than the stated purpose, and from disclosing it to any other party without further authorization. The following written statement should accompany certain disclosures:

This information has been disclosed to you from records protected by Federal confidentiality rules (42 CFR Part 2). The Federal rules prohibit you from making any further disclosure of this information unless further disclosure is expressly permitted by the written consent of the person to whom it pertains or as otherwise permitted by (42 CFR Part 2). A general authorization for the release of medical or other information is NOT sufficient for this purpose. The Federal rules restrict any use of the information to criminally investigate or prosecute any alcohol or drug abuse patient.

I specifically understand and agree that the REDISCLOSURE requirements set out above will apply to these records.

(5) **Validity.** I understand that this authorization will automatically expire one year from the date of my signature, and that I may revoke this authorization by sending a written notice to the person or entity authorized to make the disclosure described above. I agree that any release which has been made prior to revocation and which was made in reliance upon this authorization shall not constitute a breach of my rights to confidentiality.

I authorize the release of information as indicated above.

Date _____

Signature _____

Authorization To Transfer Medical Records

(1) **Patient Information**

Name _____

SSN _____

Date of Birth _____

Address _____

(2) **Authorization for Release**

I hereby authorize _____ of _____

_____, _____ _____ to
release, disclose, and deliver the medical information described below to:

Authorized Recipient:

_____

_____

_____

(3) **Specific Authorization.** I specifically authorize the release of all medical information relating to the above-named patient except I DO NOT AUTHORIZE release of information related to the areas checked below:
   ☐ Substance Abuse
   ☐ Mental Health Treatment
   ☐ HIV-AIDS

This authorization includes reports, correspondence, test results, and any other information in the records, whether generated by the authorized provider or another entity.

I do not give permission for any other use of redisclosure of this information.

Date _____

Patient _____

(4) **Redisclosure**. This release does not authorize redisclosure of medical information beyond the limits of this consent. The recipient of this information is prohibited from using the information for other than the stated purpose, and from disclosing it to any other party without further authorization. The following written statement should accompany certain disclosures:

This information has been disclosed to you from records protected by Federal confidentiality rules (42 CFR Part 2). The Federal rules prohibit you from making any further disclosure of this information unless further disclosure is expressly permitted by the written consent of the person to whom it pertains or as otherwise permitted by (42 CFR Part 2). A general authorization for the release of medical or other information is NOT sufficient for this purpose. The Federal rules restrict any use of the information to criminally investigate or prosecute any alcohol or drug abuse patient.

I specifically understand and agree that the REDISCLOSURE requirements set out above will apply to these records.

(5) **Validity.** I understand that this authorization will automatically expire one year from the date of my signature, and that I may revoke this authorization by sending a written notice to the person or entity authorized to make the disclosure described above. I agree that any release which has been made prior to revocation and which was made in reliance upon this authorization shall not constitute a breach of my rights to confidentiality.

I authorize the release of information as indicated above.

Date _____

Signature _____

Current Medical List

Patient Information

Name _____

Date of Birth _____

Medication Allergies _____

_____

_____

_____

Patient Notes

1. _____

2. _____

3. _____

4. _____

5. _____

6. _____

7. _____

8. _____

Patient Notes

Patient Notes

Patient Notes

Patient Notes

Patent Notes

Patient Notes

Patent Notes

Patient Notes

Patient Notes

Patient Notes

Surgery Information

Date of Surgery: _____

Type of Surgery: _____

Name and address of the medical institution where the surgery will be performed:

_____

_____

_____

Telephone number of medical institution: _____

Medical record Number: _____

Surgeons' name: _____

Surgeons phone number: _____

Nurse practitioner's name: _____

List any major complications:

_____

_____

_____

Suggested Records To Obtain:

- ☐ Copy of discharge summary after surgery
- ☐ Copies of all pathology reports
- ☐ Copies of all second opinions
- ☐ Copies of all imaging reports (MRI, CT, etc.) before and after surgery

If you have had more than one surgery, print out this page and have your surgeon or nurse fill in a separate page for each subsequent surgery.

Follow Up

After you have had treatment or surgery, ask your doctor(s) to fill in or provide relevant information.

Surgical Follow-Up Appointments

Healthcare Provider:	Purpose:	Frequency:

This summary of your treatment and follow-up needs was prepared by:

Healthcare Provider:	Purpose:	Frequency:

This summary of your treatment and follow-up needs was prepared by:

Healthcare Provider:	Purpose:	Frequency:

This summary of your treatment and follow-up needs was prepared by:

Healthcare Provider:	Purpose:	Frequency:

This summary of your treatment and follow-up needs was prepared by:

Patient Health Journal

Patient's Name _____

Date / Time of observation _____

Pain Level [Scale of 1-10] _____

Emotional State _____

Physical State _____

Additional Notes:

_____

_____

_____

_____

_____

_____

_____

Patient Health Journal

Patient's Name _____

Date / Time of observation _____

Pain Level [Scale of 1-10] _____

Emotional State _____

Physical State _____

Additional Notes:

Patient Health Journal

Patient's Name   _____

Date / Time of observation   _____

Pain Level [Scale of 1-10]   _____

Emotional State   _____

Physical State   _____

Additional Notes:

_____

_____

_____

_____

_____

_____

_____

_____

Patient Health Journal

Patient's Name   _____

Date / Time of observation   _____

Pain Level [Scale of 1-10]   _____

Emotional State   _____

Physical State   _____

Additional Notes:

Patient Health Journal

Patient's Name _____

Date / Time of observation _____

Pain Level [Scale of 1-10] _____

Emotional State _____

Physical State _____

Additional Notes:

_____

_____

_____

_____

_____

_____

_____

Patient Health Journal

Patient's Name   _____

Date / Time of observation   _____

Pain Level [Scale of 1-10]   _____

Emotional State   _____

Physical State   _____

Additional Notes:

_____

_____

_____

_____

_____

_____

_____

_____

Patient Health Journal

Patient's Name   _____

Date / Time of observation   _____

Pain Level [Scale of 1-10]   _____

Emotional State   _____

Physical State   _____

Additional Notes:

_____

_____

_____

_____

_____

_____

_____

_____

Patient Health Journal

Patient's Name _____

Date / Time of observation _____

Pain Level [Scale of 1-10] _____

Emotional State _____

Physical State _____

Additional Notes:

_____

_____

_____

_____

_____

_____

_____

_____

Patient Health Journal

Patient's Name   _____

Date / Time of observation   _____

Pain Level [Scale of 1-10]   _____

Emotional State   _____

Physical State   _____

Additional Notes:

_____

_____

_____

_____

_____

_____

_____

_____

Patient Health Journal

Patient's Name _____

Date / Time of observation _____

Pain Level [Scale of 1-10] _____

Emotional State _____

Physical State _____

Additional Notes:

_____

_____

_____

_____

_____

_____

_____

_____

Patient Health Journal

Patient's Name

Date / Time of observation

Pain Level [Scale of 1-10]

Emotional State

Physical State

Additional Notes:

Patient Health Journal

Patient's Name _____

Date / Time of observation _____

Pain Level [Scale of 1-10] _____

Emotional State _____

Physical State _____

Additional Notes:

_____

_____

_____

_____

_____

_____

_____

_____

Patient Health Journal

Patient's Name   _____

Date / Time of observation   _____

Pain Level [Scale of 1-10]   _____

Emotional State   _____

Physical State   _____

Additional Notes:

_____

_____

_____

_____

_____

_____

_____

_____

Patient Health Journal

Patient's Name   _____

Date / Time of observation   _____

Pain Level [Scale of 1-10]   _____

Emotional State   _____

Physical State   _____

Additional Notes:

Patient Health Journal

Patient's Name   _____

Date / Time of observation   _____

Pain Level [Scale of 1-10]   _____

Emotional State   _____

Physical State   _____

Additional Notes:

_____

_____

_____

_____

_____

_____

_____

Patient Health Journal

Patient's Name   _____

Date / Time of observation _____

Pain Level [Scale of 1-10] _____

Emotional State   _____

Physical State   _____

Additional Notes:

Patient Health Journal

Patient's Name _____

Date / Time of observation _____

Pain Level [Scale of 1-10] _____

Emotional State _____

Physical State _____

Additional Notes:

_____

_____

_____

_____

_____

_____

_____

_____

Patient Health Journal

Pat ent's Name   _____

Date / Time of observation   _____

Pain Level [Scale of 1-10]   _____

Emotional State   _____

Physical State   _____

Additional Notes:

Patient Health Journal

Patient's Name   _____

Date / Time of observation   _____

Pain Level [Scale of 1-10]   _____

Emotional State   _____

Physical State   _____

Additional Notes:

_____

_____

_____

_____

_____

_____

_____

Patient Health Journal

Patient's Name   _____

Date / Time of observation   _____

Pain Level [Scale of 1-10]   _____

Emotional State   _____

Physical State   _____

Additional Notes:

Patient Health Journal

Patient's Name   _____

Date / Time of observation   _____

Pain Level [Scale of 1-10]   _____

Emotional State   _____

Physical State   _____

Additional Notes:

_____

_____

_____

_____

_____

_____

_____

Patient Health Journal

Patient's Name   _____

Date / Time of observation   _____

Pain Level [Scale of 1-10]   _____

Emotional State   _____

Physical State   _____

Additional Notes:

_____

_____

_____

_____

_____

_____

_____

Patient Health Journal

Patient's Name   _____

Date / Time of observation   _____

Pain Level [Scale of 1-10]   _____

Emotional State   _____

Physical State   _____

Additional Notes:

_____

_____

_____

_____

_____

_____

_____

Patient Health Journal

Patient's Name   _____

Date / Time of observation   _____

Pain Level [Scale of 1-10]   _____

Emotional State   _____

Physical State   _____

Additional Notes:

Patient Health Journal

Patient's Name   _____

Date / Time of observation   _____

Pain Level [Scale of 1-10]   _____

Emotional State   _____

Physical State   _____

Additional Notes:

_____

_____

_____

_____

_____

_____

_____

_____

Patient Health Journal

Patient's Name   _____

Date / Time of observation   _____

Pain Level [Scale of 1-10]   _____

Emotional State   _____

Physical State   _____

Additional Notes:

_____

_____

_____

_____

_____

_____

_____

Patient Health Journal

Patient's Name _____

Date / Time of observation _____

Pain Level [Scale of 1-10] _____

Emotional State _____

Physical State _____

Additional Notes:

_____

_____

_____

_____

_____

_____

_____

Patient Health Journal

Patient's Name   _____

Date / Time of observation   _____

Pain Level [Scale of 1-10]   _____

Emotional State   _____

Physical State   _____

Additional Notes:

Patient Health Journal

Patient's Name   _____

Date / Time of observation   _____

Pain Level [Scale of 1-10]   _____

Emotional State   _____

Physical State   _____

Additional Notes:

_____

_____

_____

_____

_____

_____

_____

Patient Health Journal

Pat ent's Name   _____

Date / Time of observation   _____

Pain Level [Scale of 1-10]   _____

Emotional State   _____

Physical State   _____

Additional Notes:

_____

_____

_____

_____

_____

_____

_____

_____

Patient Health Journal

Patient's Name   _____

Date / Time of observation   _____

Pain Level [Scale of 1-10]   _____

Emotional State   _____

Physical State   _____

Additional Notes:

_____

_____

_____

_____

_____

_____

_____

Ovarian Cancer: Who's At Risk?

Ovarian Cancer is one of those diseases that I mentioned as not getting enough attention in my opinion.

The exact causes of Ovarian Cancer are not known; however, studies show that the following factors may increase the chances of developing this disease:

- **Family History**. First-degree relatives (mother, daughter, sister) of a woman who has had ovarian cancer are at increased risk of developing this type of cancer themselves.

- **Frequency**. The likelihood is especially high if two or more first-degree relatives have had this disease. The risk is somewhat less, but still above average, if other relatives (aunt, cousin, or grandmother) had ovarian cancer. A family history of breast or colon cancer is associated with an increased risk of developing ovarian cancer.

- **Age**. The likelihood of developing ovarian cancer increases as a woman gets older. Most ovarian cancer occurs in women over the age of 50, with the highest risk over 60.

- **Childbearing**. In fact, the more children a woman has, the less likely she is to develop ovarian cancer.

- **Personal History**. Women who have had breast or colon cancer may have a greater chance of developing ovarian cancer.

- **Fertility Drugs:** Drugs that cause a woman to ovulate may slightly increase a woman's chance to develop ovarian cancer. Researchers are studying this possible association.

- **Talc**. Some studies suggest that women who have used talc in the genital area for many years may be at increased risk of developing ovarian cancer.
- **Hormone Replacement Therapy (HRT).** Some evidence suggests that women who use HRT after menopause may slightly increase risk of developing ovarian cancer.

About 1 in 57 women in the United States will develop ovarian cancer. Most cases occur in women over the age of 50, but this disease also affects younger women.

Information taken from The American Cancer Society

About the Author

Shanna McCoy is an outstanding young woman who hails from North Little Rock, Arkansas. She has already made a lasting impact on her community in such a short time as an actress, comedian, community advocate, dancer, human-right activist, make-up artist, poet, and talented writer.

Shanna was also named Outstanding Poet of the 21st century!

Through encouragement, motivation, and tenacity, Shanna has created a formula for success through writing and motivating others. This amazing young talent was born with Cerebral Palsy and lives with a brain tumor doctors declare as inoperable.

Being a single mother of one, she is still determined not to let her many challenges and past determine the outcome of her life's destiny.

"No matter your current circumstances, you can make it. Through ambition, confidence and determination, you can live out your dreams provided you believe in yourself. It's about having faith in yourself, even when others tend to doubt your abilities."

"We Believe In Your Dreams"

Butterfly Typeface Publishing

PO Box 56193

Little Rock AR 72215

501-823-0574

info@butterflytypeface.com